"HeIP Me TaIK RiGHt"

HOW TO TEACH A CHILD TO SAY THE "L" SOUND IN 15 EASY LESSONS

by

Mirla G. Raz, M.ED., CCC

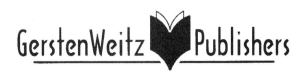

GerstenWeitz Publishers

PO. Box 5599 • Scottsdale, Arizona • 85261-5599

Other **Help Me Talk Right** books by Mirla G. Raz:

How to Correct a Child's Lisp in 15 Easy Lessons

How To Teach a Child to Say the "R" Sound in 15 Easy Lessons

Published by GerstenWeitz Publishers, P.O. Box 5599, Scottsdale, Arizona, 85261-5599

Copyright 1999 by Mirla Geclewicz Raz

Library of Congress Catalog Card Number: 98-075259

ISBN: 0-9635426-4-8

Printed in the United States of America

ACKNOWLEDGEMENTS

I would like to express my appreciation to Dannah G. Raz and Jessy Lane for the illustrations they provided for the front and back covers.

CONTENTS

INTRODUCTION TO SPEECH PATHOLOGIST

Help Me Talk Right: How to Teach a Child to Say the "L" Sound in 15 Easy Lessons is an approach to "l" correction that has made my life easier. I know it can do the same for you. This book is simple to use and follow, and it is efficient and versatile. It is a method I rely on each time I teach a child the "l"sound. I know that you will be successful in teaching the child to use the "l" sound, in conversation, approximately two months after beginning the program.

The "Help Me Talk Right" program is sequential, with each level building upon the previous one. Most of the lessons are sequenced in pairs, so that whatever the child is taught to do with initial "l" he is taught to do with final "l" in the next lesson. Built into the program are clearly defined goals, suggestions for materials that will make the sessions fun for the child, and the suggested time needed for completing each lesson. The steps for each lesson are clearly described and easy to follow. The practice sessions for each lesson reinforce what has been learned during the lesson. Like the lessons, they are easy to follow and, as a plus, they can be assigned to a parent or classroom aide. The reproducible worksheets are comprised of fun pictures and stories that the children will enjoy. A certificate of achievement is included in the manual.

Speech pathologists using the book will be able to use it as is, or make alterations, as they deem necessary. For instance, it is left to the speech pathologist's discretion to decide if the child is capable of moving through two lessons in one session.

The demand for qualified speech pathologists is far greater than the supply. As a result many of us employ aides to work under our supervision. The simplicity and efficiency of "Help Me Talk Right" make this manual perfectly suited for layperson use, under the supervision of a speech pathologist. Throughout the years that I have been a speech pathologist I have always involved parents and paraprofessionals in the therapeutic process. With this manual the nonprofessional will be able correct the "l" sound with minimal supervision. When I give this manual to a nonprofessional I am assured that the parent or paraprofessional will be carefully guided through every step of the correction of the "l" sound. Has this manual helped make my life easier? You bet it has! I know it will do the same for you.

PRELESSON

WHAT YOU NEED TO KNOW BEFORE BEGINNING THE LESSONS

The lessons you will soon begin will be easier to follow and understand after you have read the Prelesson. It is important that you read the entire Prelesson before beginning Lesson 1.
"He" and "his" have been used generically in this book.

TARGET POPULATION

This book can be used with children four years or older who do not use the "l" sound. Most children who cannot say the "l" sound tend to use a "w." Some children use a "y" for "l." So, if the child is asked to say the words "look," he will say "wook" or "yook." If the "l" is the last letter in a word the child will say "baw" instead of "ball." There are some children who will leave out the "l" when they talk. These children will say "ook" for "look." Some parents describe the child's way of talking this way as "baby talk."

The four-year-old who is capable of accomplishing the goal in Lesson 1 should be developmentally ready to say the "l" sound.

PARENTS, AIDES, AND STUDENT CLINICIANS

The nonspeech pathologist using this manual will need to work under the supervision of a speech pathologist. This is important because the layperson may have a difficult time distinguishing between an incorrectly produced "l" and one that is correctly produced. Speech pathology aides, paraprofessionals, student clinicians, and parents should consult with the supervising speech pathologist periodically as specified by her. I recommend that consultations take place after Lessons 2, 4, and 6 to make sure the child has achieved a correct "l" sound. Thereafter, with the approval of the speech pathologist, the nonprofessional can work through to Lesson 15 independently. Lesson 15 should begin with the approval of the speech pathologist. The speech pathologist should be consulted again upon completion of Lesson 15. You will be told, at that time, if some extra work is needed, or if the child has successfully completed the "l" program.

WHEN AND WHERE TO SEEK PROFESSIONAL HELP

A therapy program is started only after the problem has been identified. If you are certain the child you are working with cannot say the "l," you have identified the problem. There are, however, some children who incorrectly say other sounds as well. If a child has multiple speech errors, consult with a licensed speech pathologist (most, but not all states, license speech pathologists) or a certified speech pathologist before beginning this program. A speech pathologist, certified by the American-Speech-Language-Hearing Association, will have the letters CCC following her name and degree (example: Mirla G. Raz, M.Ed., CCC).

Your local public school should have a speech pathologist on staff. Call the school and set up an appointment to meet her. Her consultation and help should be free of charge. You can find a speech pathologist in private practice by looking in the yellow pages of your phone book, asking your child's teacher, pediatrician, a friend, or calling the American Speech-Language-Hearing Association Information Resource Center at 1-800-638-8255.

A speech pathologist will help you identify which sounds the child does not say correctly and determine which sound should be corrected first. Once the speech pathologist recommends that the child be taught how to say the "l" sound, feel free to begin Lesson One. A speech pathologist should also be consulted when any of the following occurs as you do the lessons:

- The child has completed Lessons 2, 4, 6, and 15.
- You find that you and the child do not work well together, you are continually frustrated with the progress of the child, or the child is frustrated.
- You have been unable to accomplish the goal of a lesson after trying for about two weeks.

When you are ready to consult with a speech pathologist, call and set up an appointment for a consultation. When you meet with the speech pathologist, explain what assistance you need. The problem may be addressed during the consultation, or the speech pathologist may wish to work with the child for a session or two, until the problem you have presented is resolved. Once the problem has been resolved, you can continue with the next lesson in the book.

It is important that all children have their hearing checked to rule out a hearing loss which may be causing a speech problem. Many schools – preschools and elementary – offer routine hearing screenings, as do audiologists, speech pathologists in private practice, speech clinics, and pediatricians. A hearing screening will indicate only if the child may have a hearing loss. If the hearing screening indicates a possible hearing loss or if you suspect the child may have a hearing loss, then a complete audiological evaluation, done by a licensed or certified audiologist, is recommended. An audiologist certified by the American Speech-Language-Hearing Association will have the letters CCC-A after her name and degree. (Example: Jane Smith, M.S., CCC-A).

WORKING WITH THE CHILD

It is important that anyone working with a child feel motivated to help the child. You must feel that what you are doing is valuable and will benefit the child. These feelings will be conveyed to the child through your words and words and attitude. If you feel motivated, it will be much easier to motivate the child. If you consider the child's speech lessons to be important the child will take the cue from you.

Once you have decided that you are ready to help the child, you need to tell the child that you and he will work together so that he can learn to say his "l" sound the right way. Tell him that you will be playing games and looking at pictures and that the lessons will be fun.

Praise is an important motivator. Children who are motivated try to please the adult with whom they are working. Always remember that effort, as well as success, deserves praise. Tell the child, at frequent intervals, that he is doing a fine job. Avoid using the word "No." Instead say, "Try again," or "Almost," or "Good try." Be positive and patient with the child. Impatience and/or a negative attitude will cause the child to resist doing the lessons and practice sessions.

Be alert and sensitive to the child. Motivation can wane if a child feels challenged beyond his abilities. Children will get squirmy and begin to misbehave if they can no longer sit and concentrate, or have lost interest. If a lesson time is twenty minutes and the child becomes squirmy after ten minutes, take a break for a couple of minutes to "shake the squiggles out." The child will show you he has lost interest by not paying attention, fidgeting, or misbehaving. Once the child loses interest it is best to end the session and resume the lesson later or the next day.

Maintain realistic expectations of what the child can do. After the first two or three lessons you may feel the urge to ask the child to repeat, what he just told you, using the "l" sound. For instance, the child wants to tell you about something that just happened. He uses the "w" sound instead of "l." You ask him to say the word again but with the "l" sound. <u>Avoid that temptation! Do not expect the child to use "l" in conversation because he has learned how to say "l" correctly. Do not expect him to use the "l" sound all the time until he begins Lesson 15. Do not correct him in conversation until he has begun Lesson 15.</u>

Learning to use a new "l" sound is a process that is clearly laid out in this book. It may appear simple to you, as an adult, for the child to start using "l" in conversation now that he has learned how to make the sound. In reality, it is a giant leap to go from being able to say "l" to using it all the time when talking. An unrealistic expectation will only serve to frustrate you and the child. Besides, you will find that in no time the child will be ready for Lesson 15; this lesson makes using "l" in conversation fun for the child.

Do not attempt to correct any sound but the "l" while you are working on this program. Doing so will only serve to confuse and frustrate the child. Ignore any other speech errors he makes. Focus only on the "l" sound!

It is important to make each lesson fun. Fun is motivating. You can make each lesson fun by doing things the child enjoys. For instance, use board games if the child enjoys them. Have books and crayons available if the child enjoys coloring. More is said about suggested materials later on.

Enjoy playing and working with the child. When you do the lessons, have fun!

The important points to remember when working with the child are:

- You should feel motivated to help the child.
- Praise the child frequently.
- Be sensitive and alert to the child.
- Maintain realistic expectations.
- Make the lessons fun.

LESSONS

Lessons take anywhere from 10 to 30 minutes. Do not push the child past his limit. A session that is too long can frustrate the child and you. Try to do at least one, but no more than three, lessons each week. It is very important that you follow the lessons in order. Do not skip any. Correcting a child's lisp is a process that requires learning one task before the next can be added.

Speech pathology students in clinic and speech aides may find that their scheduled appointment with the child runs longer than the time needed to complete a lesson. In other words, the child is scheduled for a half hour of therapy but the lesson is only 10 minutes long. If the child is receiving speech therapy for the "l" only and, in the your judgment, the child is capable of moving on, you may attempt to move on to the next lesson. If you decide to do more than one lesson during a therapy session, be certain that the child has met the goal of the lesson just completed, before you move on. Remember to be sensitive to the child. You want to challenge without frustrating. Stop and go back to the previous lesson if the child indicates, through responses and behavior, that he is not ready for the next lesson.

If you are a parent using this book, try to set aside the same time each day for a lesson or practice session. The child's speech sessions should be treated as ballet lessons, soccer practice, or any other scheduled activity, with its own special time during which **NOTHING ELSE IS DONE**. Do not push a lesson in when you or your child has a free moment or when you are, for instance, cooking or the child is taking a bath.

You and the child should not be distracted during the lessons and practice sessions. Make sure speech time with the child is free of common household distractions. Turn off the radio or television. Let the answering machine answer the phone for you, if you have one. If you must answer the phone, tell your caller that you cannot talk and you will call back. If there are other children at home make sure they are occupied during the lesson and practice session times. Older children can read or play in another room of the house. It may be best to do a lesson or practice session during a younger sibling's nap time.

Lessons should be done at a table, preferably a child's table. Make sure the child sits comfortably and is high enough to easily see any game, toy, and/or worksheet that is on the table.

Each lesson suggests the materials you will need, the goal of the lesson, and how long the lesson will take. The instructions for each lesson, after Lesson 1, are broken down into steps. Step One, for most lessons, will ask you to review a previous lesson or lessons. You should review the previous lesson by asking the child to do a few items of that lesson. For instance, one row of the worksheet can be done. *You do not need to do the entire worksheet when you review.*

If the child has difficulty with a lesson you will find help in the troubleshooting section, found after the practice sessions in most lessons. This section will instruct you how to make the lesson easier for the child. Refer to the troubleshooting section, if after a few attempts, the child is unable to perform the task correctly. Each lesson tells you when to refer to troubleshooting for that lesson.

MATERIALS

Activities and toys are used to make the lessons fun for the child. Prepare the materials you will be using for the lesson before you sit down with the child.

Below are examples of different activities and toys. Feel free to be innovative. Better yet, let the child decide which activity or toy he wishes to use.

Turn-taking activities: You will need turn-taking activities for Lessons 2 to 13. These materials should be appropriate for the child's age, easy for the child to follow, and allow the child and you to take turns at play. Taking a turn should be used as a reward for success. For example, the child said "l" in isolation five times, as you asked him to do. He can take a turn. Then you take a turn. Taking a turn should also be a reward for effort even if the goal has not been met. Try to finish the lesson and the turn-taking activity at the same time. As you do the lessons there will be reminders to take turns at the turn-taking activity. Some examples of turn-taking materials are:

- Board games (Candyland, Chutes and Ladders, Pizza Party, checkers, etc.)

- Coloring book and crayons (The child colors in only a segment of the picture each turn.)
- Memory Game
- Legos, blocks, logs, etc. (The child adds a few pieces at each turn to what is being built.)
- Puzzles

<u>Conversational activities</u>: These are not turn-taking activities. Instead, these materials are used to stimulate the child to talk. You will use these materials for Lesson 14. Some examples of conversational materials are:

Playing with dolls or action figures	Playing school
Talking about pictures	Reading a book together
Playing house	Playing with cars

Appendix B contains additional suggestions.

PRACTICE SESSIONS

Practice sessions are important for reinforcement and carryover of each lesson. A successful lesson must be practiced a few times before the next lesson is attempted. If the child completes a lesson on Monday, practice what was learned on Tuesday and Wednesday. A practice session is handled like a lesson except that nothing new is learned. Each lesson will tell you about the practice sessions for that lesson.

Do one practice session a day. The first practice session should be done the day after the lesson. For example, if the child does Lesson 5 on Monday, the first practice session should be done on Tuesday, the second practice session on Wednesday and so on. The next lesson can be taught after the practice sessions have been successfully completed.

An assistant can be taught how to do the practice sessions. Or, instruct the parent to do the practice sessions at home. Explain what you would like done. It is important that you also show the parent how you would like the practice session done. If the lesson calls for a turn-taking activity, ask the parent to use one as well and instruct her how to incorporate it into the practice session. Show the parent how to use the worksheet. If the lesson calls for reinforcers, explain what reinforcers are and how to use them. Show the parent how to use the worksheet. I always request that the parent bring a notebook to speech. I then write, in the notebook, what I would like the parent to do at home with the child. Using a notebook also allows me to easily and quickly refer back and see what I had asked the parent to do.

When a worksheet is needed, allow the parent to take the applicable worksheet(s) home. Request that the worksheet(s) be returned, with the notebook, for the child's next speech session.

WORKSHEETS

There are nine worksheets. They can found at the back of the book, in Appendix A. You will need a worksheet for most lessons. Each lesson will tell you which worksheet you will need for that lesson. If you like, copy the worksheet you will need and place it in front of the child before you begin the lesson. Save each worksheet. You will be using many of them for lessons further on in the book.

PRAISE, REWARDS, AND REINFORCEMENTS

Praise is extremely important. The child will know he is successful when he is praised. Because praise is so important, there will be frequent reminders, in each lesson, to praise the child. Praise comes in many forms. It can be verbal, as when you say, "Great work!" or "What a good 'l!'" Parents can use hugs and kisses accompanied by verbal praise.

- Be generous with praise.
- Avoid showing frustration, yelling, or punishing the child if he is
  having difficulty with a lesson. Patience will pay off.

Rewards and reinforcements will be explained in the applicable lessons.

CHECKLISTS

The last two pages of this Prelesson contain two checklists, the Prelesson Checklist and the Progress Checklist. Read them over before you begin. The Prelesson Checklist goes over important points discussed in the Prelesson. The Progress Checklist will help you keep track of the lessons completed.

PRELESSON CHECKLIST

Place a check on each line.

☆_____I have explained, to the child, that I will help him learn to say the "l" correctly.

☆_____I will be patient and sensitive as I work with the child.

☆_____I know what to do when the child is no longer interested in continuing the session.

☆_____I will set aside a specific time of day, each day, to work on the lessons and practice sessions.

☆_____I will use praise often as I work with the child.

☆_____I will make the lessons and practice sessions fun.

LET'S START LESSON ONE!

PROGRESS CHECKLIST

(Use this checklist to keep track of the child's progress.)

Lesson	Completed (✓)	Practice Session (cross out as completed)	
1		1 2	Good job. You are ready for the next lesson.
2		1 2	Move on to Lesson 3.
3		1 2	Good work! Moving right along.
4		1 2	Ready for words.
5		1 2 3	Nice work!
6		1 2 3	Let's pair in the next lesson.
7		1 2 3	Keep up the good work.
8		1 2 3	More than halfway through!
9		1 2	Sentences next. No problem.
10		1 2	Great job!
11		1 2	Getting close to the end.
12		1 2 3	The final stretch.
13		1 2 3	The next-to-last lesson is next.
14		1 2 3 4 5	The light at the end of the tunnel.
		Home Program	
15		60 pennies 10 nickels	Congratulations! You did it!

TONGUE POSITIONING

 GOAL
> You will teach the child to lift his tongue into the correct "l" (shown hereafter as lllll or "luh") position

 MATERIALS
> Mirror
> Worksheet 1
> Marker or crayon

 LESSON TIME
> 10 minutes

WHAT TO DO

Step One　　Sit next to the child. Place the mirror in front of you and the child. Look in the mirror, with the child, and say "Look at my tongue. Watch me lift my tongue and put it right behind my front teeth." Show the child how you lift your tongue and place the tongue tip right behind your top front teeth (see Figure A). Your mouth should be open wide enough for the child to see your tongue movement. Demonstrate this for the child again.

⇩　　　⇩　　　⇩　　　⇩　　　⇩

Step Two　　Now tell the child it is his turn to lift his tongue just as he saw you do it. As you both look in the mirror, open your mouth and lift your tongue tip to the correct position and watch the child as he does it. Praise him. Now say to the child, "Let's practice lifting our tongues five times. Every time you lift your tongue behind your front teeth you will color a happy face in one of the circles" (Worksheet 1). Praise the child, and allow him to color a happy face in a circle, after each successful attempt. See Trouble-shooting if the child has difficulty raising his tongue tip to the correct position.

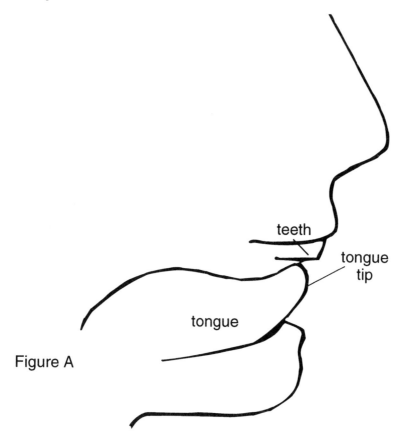

teeth

tongue tip

tongue

Figure A

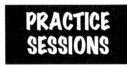

Repeat this lesson twice a day until you feel the child is ready to move on to Lesson Two.

TROUBLESHOOTING:

Some children have difficulty with the concept of raising the tongue tip. You can help the child by doing one of the following:

1. Using a Q-tip or tongue depressor, lightly touch the palate just behind the child's upper front teeth. Ask the child to open his mouth and place his tongue tip on the spot that you just touched. Repeat a few times.

2. Place a small amount of jelly on his palate, just behind his upper front teeth. Tell the child to keep his mouth open and lift his tongue to lick the jelly off the top of his mouth. Repeat a few times.

Praise the child when he lifts his tongue tip.

Once the child is able to lift his tongue tip return to Step One of this lesson. If the child is unable to lift his tongue, see Alternative Method on the next page.

ALTERNATIVE METHOD

There are some children who cannot achieve a tongue lift. There is a way to help these children produce an lllll sound without lifting the tongue. This method requires that the child place his tongue in an interdental position (Figure B). This is the same position used to say the "th" sound.

Look in the mirror with the child and do the following:

1. Protrude your tongue between your front teeth. Do not bite down or put pressure on your tongue.

2. Tell the child to place his tongue between his teeth as he sees you demonstrate. Tell the child not to bite down. He is not biting down if he is able to move his tongue around as it protrudes.

3. Say lllll with your tongue between your teeth.

4. Tell the child to say lllll with you.

5. Praise the child and repeat steps 1 to 5 a few times.

If this alternative method works, the child will most likely need to use it for the lllll sound in every lesson, including Lesson 15. Eventually the child will produce lllll without protruding his tongue.

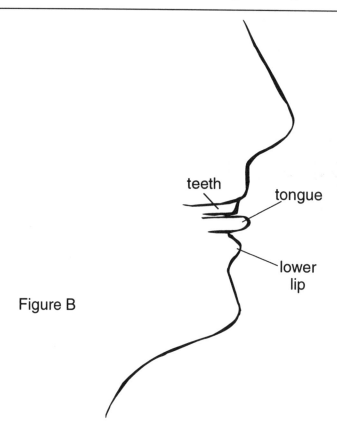

Figure B

PRODUCING THE LLLLL SOUND

GOAL

You will teach the child how to make the lllll sound.

MATERIALS

Mirror
Turn-taking activity

LESSON TIME

15 minutes

WHAT TO DO

Step One   Review what the child has learned in Lesson 1. If you used the Alternative Method, review it and skip Step Two below. However, do Step Three.

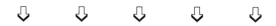

Step Two   Place the mirror in front of you and the child. Tell the child to listen carefully and watch you. Open your mouth, raise your tongue tip to your palate just behind your front teeth and say, lllll. Concentrate on making the lllll sound by holding your tongue tip behind your upper front teeth for now. Repeat a few times.

Ask the child to look in the mirror. Then ask him to say, lllll with you. Together say lllll a few times. Allow the child to take a turn at the activity he selected. Then you take a turn. If the child makes a sound that sounds more like "lwuh" or "wuh" see Troubleshooting. If his lllll sounds good continue on to Step Three.

Step Three   Ask the child to say lllll by himself. If he is successful ask him to say it five times in a row. Take turns at the activity.

The child will need to practice saying lllll over the next two days before you move on to the next lesson. The idea is to carryover and reinforce correct production of the lllll sound. Practice Session 1 is done the day after the lesson. Practice Session 2 is done the day after Practice Session 1. As much time should be spent on the Practice Sessions as was spent on the lesson. Repeat the lesson once in the morning and once in the afternoon.

Practice Session 1

You will need about 10 pennies, chips, or anything else that can be used as a reinforcer.

Practice Session 2

Face the child so that he can see your mouth. Tell the child that you are going to play the "Catch Me" game. Tell him that you will try to trick him and he has to catch you. Tell the child that each time he catches you he will win a penny.

Tell the child that sometimes you will say lllll the right way with your tongue tip up (demonstrate) or as you did in the Alternative Method. When you say lllll the right way he should say, "Good talking." If he catches you saying lllll, he will win a penny. Then tell him that sometimes you will say lllll the wrong way. Tell the child that instead of lllll you will say, lwuh (demonstrate). When you say, lwuh he has to catch you. When he catches you he says, "Wrong." Tell the child that he will win a penny when he catches you saying lllll the wrong way. When he catches you saying lwuh ask him to help you say it correctly. Then say lllll or together. Do a couple of practice trials with the child, using pennies, so that you are sure he understands what he has to do.

Switch roles after the child has caught you a few times. This time the child tries to trick you. The child will enjoy giving you pennies for catching him say lllll correctly and incorrectly. Play "Catch Me" for about ten minutes.

TROUBLESHOOTING:

Some children do not make a clear lllll sound because they round their lips which results in a "w" sound. You can help the child avoid the "w" by doing the following:

1. Look in the mirror with the child. Ask the child to watch you.

2. Open you mouth, lift your tongue tip to your palate behind your front teeth, and then pull your lips back into a smile. Make sure your mouth and tongue remain in position as you smile. Demonstrate this a couple more times.

3. Tell the child it is his turn to lift his tongue and then smile as his tongue stays behind his front teeth. Once the child has opened his mouth and lifted his tongue say, "Now keep your tongue up and smile." Have the child do this five times.

4. Continue to look in the mirror with the child. Open your mouth, lift your tongue tip, hold the smile as you say, lllll. Repeat a few times.

5. Tell the child it is his turn to say lllll while he smiles. Instruct him to open his mouth, lift his tongue tip, smile, keep smiling as says lllll. Have the child do this ten times in a row.

Return to Step One in the Lesson once the child is able to correctly produce lllll.

Do not ask or expect the child to use lllll in conversation yet.

INITIAL LLLLL IN SIMPLE SYLLABLES

 GOAL

You will teach the child to use initial lllll in combination with a vowel (the lllll sound will be followed by a vowel sound).

 MATERIALS

 Mirror
Turn-taking activity

 LESSON TIME

20 minutes

WHAT TO DO

Step One   Look in the mirror with the child. Ask the child to say lllll. If he is able to say lllll five times, continue on to Step Two. If he is unable to say the lllll five times, review Lesson 2 until the child is able to say lllll five times. Do not move on to Step Two until the child is able to say lllll five times in a row.

⇩   ⇩   ⇩   ⇩   ⇩

Step Two   You will now help the child learn to use lllll in combination with different vowel sounds. The child will be combining lllll with:

"a" as in "ape." This "a" will be shown as $\bar{a}$.
"e" as in "eat." This "e" will be shown as $\bar{e}$.
"i" as in "ice." This "i" will be shown as $\bar{i}$.
"o" as in "old." This "o" will be shown as $\bar{o}$.
"o" as in "shoe." This "o" will be shown as $\overline{oo}$.

Ask the child to say: l$\bar{a}$, l$\bar{e}$, l$\bar{i}$, l$\bar{o}$, l$\overline{oo}$. If the child correctly says the lllll with each vowel, praise him and allow him to take a turn at the turn-taking activity. Repeat this step until the turn-taking activity is completed or the child has indicated he is no longer interested in continuing. See Troubleshooting if the child is unable to produce a clear lllll when producing these syllables.

PRACTICE SESSIONS

Practice Sessions 1 & 2   The child may select a turn-taking activity if he wishes. Ask the child to repeat each lllll + vowel combination after you, just as was done for the lesson. Praise the child for a job well done. If you are playing a game, allow him to take a turn at the game after he has repeated two or three lllll + vowel combinations.

TROUBLESHOOTING:

Some children have difficulty making the transition from the lllll to the next sound. You can make this easier for the child by inserting a pause between the lllll and the vowel that follows.

Ask the child to hold his lips back in a smile and say the lllll sound then the ā sound. Demonstrate by doing the following: protract your lips, lift your tongue tip behind your top front teeth, (or protrude your tongue between your teeth) say the lllll sound, pause, then say ā. Ask the child to do the same. Praise him for a successful attempt.

You will now ask the child to say the lllll sound with the other vowel sounds. You will say each lllll sound, pause, then one of the vowel sounds. The child will repeat what you have just said and the way you presented it. Continue until you have combined, and the child has repeated, each lllll + vowel combination. Remember to praise the child. He can take a turn at the activity each time he repeats an lllll + vowel series. As this step becomes easier for the child, decrease the pause time between the lllll sound and the vowel. Your child will be ready to return to Step Two once he can say: lā, lē, lī, lō, lo͞o.

Do not ask or expect the child to use lllll in conversation yet.

FINAL LLLLL IN SIMPLE SYLLABLES

GOAL

You will teach the child to use a vowel sound in combination with final lllll (the lllll sound will follow the vowel sound).

MATERIALS

Mirror
Turn-taking activity

LESSON TIME

20 minutes

WHAT TO DO

Step One

Review initial lllll simple syllables learned in Lesson 3. Praise the child for a job well done and allow him to take a turn at the activity selected. Move on to Step Two. If the child has difficulty using initial lllll in simple syllables continue to review Lesson 3. You may, however, continue on to Step Two below.

⇩　　　⇩　　　⇩　　　⇩　　　⇩

Step Two

You will now help the child learn to use final lllll in combination with different vowel sounds. The child will be combining lllll with:

"a" as in "ape." This "a" will be shown as $\overline{a}$.
"e" as in "eat." This "e" will be shown as $\overline{e}$.
"i" as in "ice." This "i" will be shown as $\overline{i}$.
"o" as in "old." This "o" will be shown as $\overline{o}$.
"o" as in "shoe." This "o" will be shown as $\overline{oo}$.

Look in the mirror with the child. Ask the child to say:
$\overline{a}$lllll, $\overline{e}$lllll, $\overline{i}$lllll, $\overline{o}$lllll, $\overline{oo}$lllll. If the child correctly says the lllll after each vowel, praise him and allow him to take a turn at the turn-taking activity. Repeat this step until the activity is completed or the child has indicated he is no longer interested in continuing. If the child is unable to say the lllll when producing these syllables, continue on to Step Three.

⇩　　　⇩　　　⇩　　　⇩　　　⇩

Step Three
optional

This optional step teaches the child to say the final lllll as "luh." It is recommended that this step be included if the child's production of final lllll, in Step Two, is not clear. It is also suggested that you include this step because the final lllll sound can be difficult for children to hear and produce. Producing it as "luh" helps the child recognize that the word ends in an lllll. Too often, attempting to teach final lllll without attaching the "uh" results in the continued omission of lllll or the substitution of "w." It is suggested that "luh" be used in Lessons 6 and 8, where final lllll is targeted, unless the child produces the final lllll clearly in those lessons. If the final lllll is not clear, then adding "luh" will be important (Note: the child, on his own, will drop the "uh" but retain a clear lllll during Lesson 15, if not sooner.)

Ask the child to watch you as you say lllll. Lift your tongue tip behind your upper front teeth. As you say the lllll sound drop your tongue so that you say, "luh". Repeat three times. Next ask the child to say "luh" with you as you both look in the mirror. If the child is successful, ask him to say it alone five times. Take turns at the turn-taking activity.

Look in the mirror with the child. Ask the child to say: āluh, ēluh, īluh, ōluh, ōōluh. If the child correctly says the "luh" after each vowel, praise him and allow him to take a turn at the turn-taking activity. Continue combining the vowels with "luh" until the activity is completed or the child has indicated he is no longer interested in continuing. If he is not successful, *see* Troubleshooting.

PRACTICE SESSIONS

The child may select a turn-taking activity if he wishes. Ask the child to repeat the vowel + lllll or vowel + luh combinations after you, just as you did for the lesson. Praise him for a job well done. If a turn-taking activity was selected, allow him to take a turn at the turn-taking activity.

Practice Sessions 1 & 2

TROUBLESHOOTING:

Some children have difficulty making the transition from any sound to the lllll sound. You can make this easier for the child by inserting a pause between the vowel sound and the lllll.

Ask the child to say the ā then luh. Demonstrate this by doing the following: Say the ā, pause, pull your lips back into a smile, lift your tongue tip behind your top front teeth and say, "Luh." Ask the child to do the same. Praise him for a successful attempt and allow the child to take a turn.

You will now ask the child to combine the other vowels with luh. You will say the vowel sound, pause, smile, lift your tongue and say, "Luh". The child will repeat what you have just said and the way you presented it. Continue until you have combined, and the child has repeated, each vowel + luh combination. Remember to praise the child. He can take a turn at the activity each time he repeats a vowel + luh series. As this step becomes easier for the child, decrease the pause time between the vowel and the luh. Your child will be ready to return to Step Two once he can say āluh, ēluh, īluh, ōluh, ōōluh without the pause.

Do not ask or expect the child to use lllll in conversation yet.

INITIAL LLLLL IN SIMPLE WORDS

 GOAL

You will teach the child how to say the initial lllll sound in simple words.

  MATERIALS

Worksheet 2
Turn-taking activity

 LESSON TIME

20 minutes

WHAT TO DO

Step One   Review initial and final simple syllables in Lessons 3 and 4. Praise the child for a job well done. Allow him to take a turn at the activity selected. Move on to Step Two. If the child has difficulty using initial lllll in simple syllables, return to Lesson 3. Do not continue with Lesson 5 until the child successfully completes Lesson 3. If the child has difficulty with final lllll in simple syllables, continue to work on Lesson 4. You may, however, continue on to Step Two below.

⇩   ⇩   ⇩   ⇩   ⇩

Step Two   You will now help the child use initial lllll in simple words. Place Worksheet 2 in front of the child. Worksheet 2 is made up of pictures whose names begin with the lllll sound.

You name the first picture. The child names the picture after you. If he has named the picture using a correct lllll, praise him. Do the next two pictures. Allow the child to take a turn at the turn-taking activity after he has named three pictures. You also take a turn. You continue in this way until you and the child have named each picture. Remember to take turns at the selected activity. Review the sheet a second time, taking turns at the selected activity. Go over the sheet a third time, but this time you point to each picture and the child tries to name it on his own. If he has difficulty with a picture you name it and he will name it after you.

See Troubleshooting if the child says the "w" or "y" sound for lllll when repeating each word or has difficulty repeating initial lllll in simple words.

PRACTICE SESSIONS

Practice Session 1   Look through magazines, newspapers, or catalogues with the child. Look for ten pictures that begin with lllll followed by a vowel (a, e, i, o, u). As you and the child find initial lllll pictures do the following:

1. You name the picture.
2. The child names the picture.
3. The child cuts and pastes the picture on a piece of paper. (Some children may need assistance with cutting and pasting.)

4. The child names each picture using a correct lllll.

Praise the child for a job well done.

Practice Sessions 2 & 3

Use Worksheet 2 and the pasted pictures. Place Worksheet 2 and the pasted pictures in front of the child. Point to an initial lllll picture and ask the child to name it. Continue pointing, as the child names pictures, until the child has completed naming the pasted pictures and the pictures on Worksheet 2, or the child indicates he has lost interest. A variation of the above is asking the child to point to and name any three pictures he wishes. Continue in this way until the activity is completed or the child indicates that he has lost interest.

TROUBLESHOOTING:

Some children have difficulty connecting the lllll into a word. The child is accustomed to naming words with his old sound and to say the word a different way may be confusing. You can help the child get over this difficulty by using a pause. As you say each word, separate the lllll from the rest of the word. In other words, say, "Llllll", wait 2 seconds and say, "Ion." for "lion." The child repeats the word with the pause. Below are examples for a few more words:

lllll	(2 second pause)	"eopard" for "leopard"
lllll	(2 second pause)	"obster" for "lobster"
lllll	(2 second pause)	"ady" for "ladybug"

Continue in this way for all the pictures. Gradually reduce the pause time until the child can name each picture without a pause. Once this occurs return to Step One. Do not be concerned if the child needs to stay in Troubleshooting a few days. He can still do the Practice Sessions using the pause and later without the pause.

Do not ask or expect the child to use lllll in conversation yet.

FINAL LLLLL IN SIMPLE WORDS

 GOAL

You will teach the child how to say the final lllll sound in simple words.

 MATERIALS

Worksheet 3
Turn-taking activity

 LESSON TIME

20 minutes

WHAT TO DO

<u>Step One</u>

Review initial lllll in simple words in Lesson 5. Praise the child for a job well done. Allow him to take a turn at the activity selected. Move on to Step Two. If the child has difficulty using final lllll in simple syllables, return to Lesson 4. Do not move on to Step Two until the child is successful at Lesson 4. If the child has difficulty using initial lllll in simple words continue to work on Lesson 5. You may, however, continue on to Step Two.

⇩　　　⇩　　　⇩　　　⇩　　　⇩

<u>Step Two</u>

You will now help the child use final lllll in simple words. Place Worksheet 3 in front of the child. Worksheet 3 is made up of pictures whose names end with the lllll sound.

You name the first picture. The child names the picture after you. Make sure that the child lifts his tongue behind his top front teeth for the final lllll sound. Or, model the word with "luh" at the end and ask the child to repeat it. For example, for "ball" you say, "Balluh." The child repeats, "Balluh." Allow the child to take a turn at the turn-taking activity after he has named three pictures. You also take a turn. Continue in this way until you and the child have named each picture. Remember to take turns at the selected activity. Review the sheet a second time, taking turns at the selected activity. Go over the sheet a third time, but this time you point to each picture and the child tries to name it on his own. If he has difficulty with a picture, you name it and ask him to name it after you.

See Troubleshooting if the child says the "w" sound for the lllll when repeating each word or has difficulty repeating final lllll in simple words.

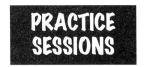

Look through magazines, newspapers, or catalogues, with the child. Look for ten pictures that end in the lllll sound. As you and the child find final lllll pictures do the following:
1. You name the picture.
2. The child names the picture.
3. The child cuts and pastes the picture on a piece of paper. (Some children may need assistance with cutting and pasting.)
4. The child names each picture, using a correct lllll. Praise the child for a job well done.

**Practice
Session 1**

Use Worksheet 3 and the pasted pictures. Place the worksheet and pasted pictures in front of the child. Point to a final lllll picture and ask the child to name it. Continue pointing, as the child names pictures, until the child has completed naming the pasted pictures and the pictures on Worksheet 3 or the child indicates he has lost interest. Praise the child for a job well done. A variation of the above is asking the child to point to and name any three pictures he wishes. Continue in this way until the activity is completed or the child indicates that he has lost interest.

**Practice
Sessions 2 & 3**

TROUBLESHOOTING

Some children have difficulty connecting the lllll into a word. The child is accustomed to naming words with his old sound and to say the word a different way may be confusing. You can help the child get over this difficulty by using a pause. Use Worksheet 3. As you say each word, separate the lllll from the rest of the word. In other words, say the word without the lllll at the end, wait two seconds, then say, "Lllll" or "Luh." For example, for the word "bell" say, "Be," wait two seconds then say, "Lllll" or "Luh." The child repeats the word with the pause. Below are examples for a few more words:

app	(2 second pause)	lllll or luh for "apple"
popsic	(2 second pause)	lllll or luh for "popsicle"
kett	(2 second pause)	lllll or luh for "kettle"

Continue in this way for all the pictures on the worksheet. Gradually reduce the pause time until the child can name each picture without a pause. Once this occurs return to Step One. Do not be concerned if the child needs to stay in Troubleshooting a few days. He can still do the Practice Sessions using the pause and later without the pause.

Do not ask or expect the child to use lllll in conversation yet.

PAIRING INITIAL LLLLL IN SIMPLE WORDS

 GOAL

You will teach the child how to pair two words that begin with the lllll sound.

  MATERIALS

Worksheet 2
Turn-taking activity

 LESSON TIME

20 minutes

WHAT TO DO

Step One   Review initial and final words in Lessons 5 and 6. Praise the child for a job well done. Allow him to take a turn at the activity selected. Move on to Step Two. If the child has difficulty using initial lllll in simple words return to Lesson 5. Do not move on to Step Two until your child is successful at Lesson 5. If the child has difficulty using final lllll in simple words continue to do Lesson 6 until the child is successful. You may, however, move on to Step Two, if the child succeeded in completing Lesson 5.

⇩   ⇩   ⇩   ⇩   ⇩

Step Two   You will now help the child pair initial simple words. Place Worksheet 2 in front of the child. Each picture on the sheet will be paired with one of the following initial lllll words: *look, like, let, leave.* As you point to the pictures in each row you will say:

[First Row]: *look lion, look leopard, look lobster, look ladybug.*
[Second Row]: *like lizard, like lamb, like leaf, like lemon.*
[Third Row]: *let lamp, let light, let luggage, let lock.*
[Fourth Row]: *leave log, leave love, leave loaf, leave lunch.*

Begin with the first row. Point to the first picture. Say the paired words. Ask the child to say what you said. Make sure he uses initial lllll in both words of the pair. You and the child take turns at the turn-taking activity. Move on to Step Three if the child pairs without difficulty. See Troubleshooting if the child has difficulty saying lllll in both words.

⇩   ⇩   ⇩   ⇩   ⇩

Step Three   Now point to each picture and say the word pairs for each picture in the rest of the row. The child will repeat the word pair for each picture after you. Take turns at the turn-taking activity after you complete the row.

Move on to the second row of pictures. Point and say the word pair for each picture. The child will repeat the word pair for each picture after you. Take turns at the turn-taking activity after you complete the row. Do rows three and four as you did rows one and two. Remember to praise the child for a job well done.

Practice the word pairs using the worksheet, just as you did for the lesson. The child may want to say the paired words on his own without repeating them after you. Excellent. Actually, you might encourage him to do so. Allow the child to decide whether or not he wishes to select a turn-taking activity. Some children enjoy doing the worksheet alone. You can even try putting a reinforcer such as a poker chip, raisin, M&M, or penny on each picture that the child correctly completes. Pennies, poker chips, etc., on the pictures allow the child to see how well he is doing. Do not put a reinforcer on a picture that was difficult for the child. After he completes the sheet go back to the pictures that do not have a reinforcement and practice those. Place a reinforcer on each picture as the child succeeds saying the word pair. Praise the child for a job well done.

Practice Session 1

Practice word pairs using the worksheet. However, this time switch the words *look, like, let,* and *leave* to different rows. In other words, pair each picture in the first row with, for example, the word *leave.* You will say *leave lion, leave leopard,* and so on. Once again the child can select a turn-taking activity or he may choose to do the sheet alone. Pennies, M&Ms, etc., may also be used as in Practice Session 1. Praise the child for a job well done.

Practice Session 2

The child can do Practice Session 3 with or without a turn-taking activity.

Practice Session 3

This session the child will start by selecting any three pictures, on Worksheet 2, for pairing. He will point to each picture and pair that picture with any other word that begins with lllll. He can use *look, like, let* and *leave* if he chooses. Or, he may choose to think of his own pairing word, such as "listen." Thus, the child may point to "lion," pair it with "listen" and say, "Listen lion." After he has paired the first three pictures, he selects another pictures for word pairing. This time he uses a different pairing word, such as "lose" to pair with the picture he has selected. Continue in this fashion, three pictures at a time, until all the pictures on the worksheet have been paired. Praise the child for a job well done.

TROUBLESHOOTING

Some children have difficulty remembering to use lllll twice. You can help the child get over this difficulty by saying each word of the pair individually. In other words you say the first word of the pair and the child repeats that word. Then say the second word of the pair and ask the child to repeat that word. The word pairs for each row of the worksheet are found under Step Two.

Below is an example of how you should present the pairs in Troubleshooting:

> You say: *Look*
> The child says: *Look*
> You say: *Lion*
> The child says: *Lion*

You can do Step Two and Practice Sessions 1 and 2 with the child. Just remember that the child repeats the first word of the pair before you say the second word of the pair. Praise him for a job well done. When you feel the child is ready, ask him to repeat an entire word pair. If he is successful, do Step Two and the Practice Sessions as written. If the child has difficulty repeating the word pair stay in Troubleshooting until the child is able to repeat two initial lllll words together.

Do not ask or expect the child to use lllll in conversation yet.

PAIRING FINAL LLLLL IN SIMPLE WORDS

 GOAL

You will teach the child how to pair two words that end with the lllll sound.

 MATERIALS

 Worksheet 3
Turn-taking activity

 LESSON TIME

20 minutes

WHAT TO DO

Step One   Review final words in Lesson 6 and initial word pairs in Lesson 7. Praise the child for a job well done. Allow him to take a turn at the activity selected. Move on to Step Two. If the child has difficulty using final lllll in simple words return to Lesson 6. Do not move on to Step Two until the child is successful at Lesson 6. If the child has difficulty using initial lllll in word pairs continue to do Lesson 7 until the child is successful. You may, however, move on to Step Two, if the child succeeded in completing Lesson 6.

⇩   ⇩   ⇩   ⇩   ⇩

Step Two   Your will now help the child pair final words. Place Worksheet 3 in front of the child. Each picture on the sheet will be paired with one of the following final lllll words: *tell, sell, pull, call.* As you point to the pictures in each row you will say:

[First Row]: *tell apple, tell popsicle, tell kettle, tell mule.*
[Second Row]: *sell turtle, sell shell, sell school, sell scale.*
[Third Row]: *pull bottle, pull candle, pull ball, pull pencil.*
[Fourth Row]: *call tool, call bell, call bicycle, call mail.*

Begin with the first row. Point to the first picture. Say the paired words. Ask the child to say what you said. Make sure he uses final lllll or luh in each word of the pair. You and the child take turns at the turn-taking activity. Continue on to Step Three if the child pairs without difficulty. See Troubleshooting if the child has difficulty using lllll in both words.

⇩   ⇩   ⇩   ⇩   ⇩

Step Three   Now point to each picture and say the word pairs for each picture in the rest of the row. The child will repeat the word pair for each picture after you. Take turns at the turn-taking activity after you complete the row.

Move on to the second row of pictures. Point and say the word pair for each picture. The child will repeat the word pair for each picture after you. Take turns at the turn-taking activity after you complete the row. Do rows three and four as you did rows one and two.

**Practice
Session 1**

Practice the word pairs using the picture sheet just as you did for the lesson. The child may want to say the paired words on his own, without repeating them after you. Excellent. Actually, you might encourage him to do so. Allow the child to decide whether or not he wishes to select a turn-taking activity. Some children enjoy doing the worksheet alone. You can even try putting a reinforcer such as poker chip, raisin, M & M, or penny on each picture that the child correctly completes. Do not put a reinforcer on a picture that was difficult for the child. After he completes the sheet go back to the pictures that do not have a reinforcer and practice those. Place a poker chip or penny, etc., on each picture as the child succeeds saying the word pair. Praise the child for a job well done.

**Practice
Session 2**

Practice word pairs using the worksheet. However, this time switch the words *tell, sell, pull* and *call* to different rows. In other words, pair each picture in the first row with, for example, the word *call*. You will say *call apple, call popsicle, call kettle, call mule.* You will use a different first word for rows two, three and four. Once again the child can select a turn-taking activity if he chooses or do the sheet alone. Pennies, raisins, etc., may also be used as in Practice Session 1. Praise the child for a job well done.

**Practice
Session 3**

The child can do Practice Session 3 with or without a turn-taking activity.

This session your child will select any three pictures, on Worksheet 3, for pairing. He will point to each picture and pair that picture with any word he selects that ends in lllll. He can use *tell, sell, pull,* and *call* if he chooses. Or he may choose to think of his own pairing word, such as "will." Thus the child may point to "apple," pair it with "will" and say, "Will apple." After he has paired the first three pictures, he selects another three pictures for word pairing. This time he uses a different pairing word to pair with the picture. Continue in this fashion, three pictures at a time, until all the pictures on the worksheet have been paired. Praise the child for a job well done.

TROUBLESHOOTING

Some children have difficulty remembering to use lllll twice. You can help the child get over this difficulty by saying each word of the pair individually. In other words, you say the first word of the pair and the child repeats that word. Then say the second word of the pair and ask the child to repeat that word. The word pairs for each row of the worksheet are found under Step Two.

Below is an example of how you should present the pairs in Troubleshooting:

You say: *Tell* or *telluh*
The child says: *Tell* or *telluh*
You say: *Apple* or *appluh*
The child says: *Apple* or *appluh*

You can do Step Two and Practice Sessions 1 and 2 with the child. Just remember that the child repeats the first word of the pair before you say the second word of the pair. When you feel the child is ready, ask him to repeat an entire word pair. If he is successful, do Step Two and the Practice Sessions as written. If the child has difficulty repeating the word pair, stay in Troubleshooting until the child is able to repeat two final lllll words together.

Do not ask or expect the child to use lllll in conversation yet.

MEDIAL LLLLL IN SIMPLE WORDS

 GOAL

You will teach the child to use lllll in the middle of words.

  MATERIALS

Worksheet 4
Turn-taking activity

 LESSON TIME

20 minutes

WHAT TO DO

Step One   Review Lessons 7 and 8. Praise the child for a job well done. Allow him to take a turn at the activity selected.

⇩   ⇩   ⇩   ⇩   ⇩

Step Two   You will now help the child use the medial lllll sound in words. Place Worksheet 4 in front of the child. You name the first picture. The child names the picture after you. Allow the child to take a turn at the turn-taking activity selected after he has named three pictures after you. You also take a turn. Continue naming and taking turns at the activity until you and the child have named each picture. Review the sheet a second time, taking turns at the selected activity. Praise the child for a job well done. See Troubleshooting if the child uses a "w" sound instead of lllll when repeating each word or has difficulty repeating lllll in simple words.

PRACTICE SESSIONS

Practice Session 1   Practice medial words using the picture sheet just as you did for the lesson. Allow the child to decide whether or not he wishes to select a turn-taking activity. Or, the child may decide to place a reinforcer such as a poker chip, raisin, M&M, or penny on each picture that he correctly names. Do not allow the child to put a poker chip, etc., on a picture whose name he said incorrectly. After he completes the sheet go back to the pictures that do not have a reinforcer on them and practice those. Place a reinforcer on each picture as the child successfully says the medial lllll word. Praise the child for a job well done.

Practice Session 2   The child can do Practice Session 2 with or without a turn-taking activity.

This session the child will select any three pictures. He will point to each picture and name it using a correct lllll. Praise him for a job well done. The child will continue in this fashion until all the pictures on the worksheet have been named.

TROUBLESHOOTING

Some children have difficulty making the transition from lllll to the next sound. You can help the child get over this difficulty by separating the portion of the word containing the "l" from the preceding syllable(s). By doing this the lllll is produced as an initial lllll sound. In other words, you say the first part of the word and the child repeats that part. Then say the second part containing the lllll and ask the child to repeat that part.

Words are broken down as follows:

balloon	ba	lloon
umbrella	umbre	lla
envelope	enve	lope
telephone	te	lephone
television	te	levision
elephant	e	lephant
alligator	a	lligator
watermelon	waterme	lon
calendar	ca	lendar
dollar	do	llar
violin	vio	lin
broccoli	brocco	li
island	is	land
helicopter	he	licopter
stapler	stap	ler
ballet	ba	llet

Complete Worksheet 4 with the child repeating one part at a time. Remember to take turns at the turn-taking activity after each group of three pictures. Praise the child for a job well done. Stay in Troubleshooting until the child is able to say medial lllll in a word without breaking it down into two parts.

You can do Practice Sessions 1 and 2 with the child. Just remember that the child repeats each syllable separately after you until you feel he is ready to use medial lllll without a word breakdown. When you feel the child is ready, return to Step Two of the lesson.

Do not ask or expect the child to use lllll in conversation yet.

INITIAL LLLLL IN SIMPLE SENTENCES

 GOAL

You will teach the child to use initial lllll in simple sentences.

  MATERIALS

Worksheet 2
Turn-taking activity

 LESSON TIME

20 minutes

WHAT TO DO

Step One   Review initial and final pairs and medial words in Lessons 7, 8, and 9. Praise the child for a job well done. Allow him to take a turn at the activity selected. Move on to Step Two. If the child has difficulty using initial lllll in pairs return to Lesson 7. Do not move on to Step Two until the child is successful at Lesson 7. If the child has difficulty using final lllll in pairs or medial lllll in simple words continue to do those lessons until the child is successful. You may, however, move on to Step Two, if the child succeeded in completing Lesson 7.

⇩   ⇩   ⇩   ⇩   ⇩

Step Two   You will now help the child use the word pairs of Lesson 7 in simple sentences. Place Worksheet 2 in front of the child. You will work a row at a time as you did in Lesson 7. (Some of the sentences will not make sense. That is okay. Right now our goal is for the child to begin using the lllll sound in sentences.) Each sentence will begin with the word "I" plus a verb. You will say the following:

> [First Row]: *I look at the lion; I look at the leopard; I look at the lobster; I look at the ladybug.*
> [Second Row]: *I like the lizard; I like the lamb; I like the leaf; I like the lemon.*
> [Third Row]: *I let the lamp; I let the light; I let the luggage; I let the lock.*
> [Fourth Row]: *I leave the log; I leave the love; I leave the loaf; I leave the lunch.*

Begin with the first row of pictures. Point to the first picture. Say the sentence for that picture. Ask the child to say what you said. Make sure he uses initial lllll in each word starting with lllll. Praise the child for a job well done. Take turns at the turn-taking activity. Continue on to Step Three if the child repeats the sentence without difficulty. See Troubleshooting if the child has difficulty using lllll in simple sentences.

⇩   ⇩   ⇩   ⇩   ⇩

Now point and say the sentence for each picture in the rest of the row. The child will repeat the sentence for each picture after you. Praise the child for a job well done. Take turns at the turn-taking activity. Continue doing rows two, three and four in the same way.

PRACTICE SESSIONS

Practice the simple sentences using the worksheet just as you did for the lesson. The child may want to say the sentences on his own, without repeating them after you. Excellent. Actually, you might encourage him to do so. Allow the child to decide whether or not he wishes to select a turn-taking activity or use reinforcers (pennies, poker chips, etc). Once the child has completed the sheet go back and practice any sentences that were difficult for him.

Practice Session 1

Practice sentences using the worksheet. However, this time switch the first two words of the sentences with the other rows. In other words, say each picture in the first row with *I leave* instead of *I look*. You will say *I leave the lion, I leave the leopard, I leave the lobster, I leave the ladybug.* Switch *I look* to another row, such as row two, *I like* to row three, and *I let* to row four. You can use any first two words with any row you or the child wishes. Once again the child can select a turn-taking activity, if he chooses, or do the sheet alone. Reinforcers (pennies, M&M, etc.), may also be used. Since this is the last time you will be using this worksheet, the child can color, put a sticker or draw a happy face on each picture for which lllll was correctly said. Do not allow the child to color or put a sticker on a picture he said incorrectly. After he completes the sheet, go back to the pictures that are not colored or do not have a sticker. Practice those pictures. Allow the child to color or put a sticker or happy face on each picture as he succeeds in saying the sentence correctly. Praise him for a job well done.

Practice Session 2

TROUBLESHOOTING

Some children have difficulty remembering to use lllll in a sentence. You can help the child get over this difficulty by saying each lllll word of the sentence individually. In other words, you say, "I" and the child repeats, "I." Next say, "Look" which the child repeats. Then ask the child to repeat, "At the." Last, say the picture name, such as "lion" which the child repeats. Praise the child for a job well done.

Stay on the first picture. This time ask the child to repeat, "I look." Praise the child for a job well done. Now ask him to repeat, "At the lion." Praise him again. Tell the child that this time he will say the whole sentence after you. You slowly say, "I look at the lion." Ask the child to repeat what you just said. Praise him for a job well done. Complete the first row in this way. Return to Step Two of this lesson once the child repeats each simple sentence in the first row, in its entirety, using correct lllll in the sentences. Remember to take turns at the turn-taking activity.

If the child has difficulty repeating the entire sentence, stay with "I look," which he repeats, then "at the lion" which he repeats. Complete the worksheet in this way. Reintroduce the entire sentence, "I look at the lion," once you feel the child is ready. The child will be ready to do Step Two of this lesson once he can repeat an entire simple sentence, in its entirety, for each picture in the first row.

Do not ask or expect the child to use lllll in conversation yet.

FINAL LLLLL IN SIMPLE SENTENCES

 GOAL

You will teach the child to use final lllll in simple sentences.

 MATERIALS

Worksheet 3
Turn-taking activity

 LESSON TIME

20 minutes

WHAT TO DO

Step One   Review final pairs in Lesson 8, medial lllll in words in Lesson 9, and initial lllll in simple sentences in Lesson 10. Praise the child for a job well done. Allow him to take a turn at the activity selected. Move on to Step Two. If the child has difficulty using *final* lllll in pairs return to Lesson 8. Do not move on to Step Two until the child is successful at Lesson 8. If the child has difficulty using medial lllll in words (Lesson 9) or initial lllll in simple sentences (Lesson 10) continue to do those lessons until the child is successful. You may, however, also move on to Step Two, if the child succeeded in completing Lesson 8.

⇩   ⇩   ⇩   ⇩   ⇩

Step Two   You will now help the child use the word pairs, of Lesson 8, in simple sentences. Place Worksheet 3 in front of the child. You will work a row at a time as you did in Lesson 8. (Some of the sentences will not make sense. That is okay. Right now our goal is for the child to begin using the lllll sound in sentences.)

Look at the worksheet. You will say the following:

> [First Row]: *I tell the apple; I tell the popsicle; I tell the kettle; I tell the mule.*
> [Second Row]: *I sell the turtle; I sell the shell; I sell the school; I sell the scale.*
> [Third Row]: *I pull the bottle; I pull the candle; I pull the ball; I pull the pencil.*
> [Fourth Row]: *I call the tool; I call the bell; I call the bicycle; I call the mail.*

Begin with the first row of pictures. Point to the first picture. Say the sentence for that picture. Ask the child to say what you said. Make sure he uses final lllll or luh in each word ending with lllll. Praise the child for a job well done. Take turns at the turn-taking activity. Continue on to Step Three if the child repeats the sentence without difficulty.

See Troubleshooting if the child has difficulty using lllll in simple sentences.

Step Three

Now point and say the sentence for each picture in the rest of the row. The child will repeat the sentence for each picture. Praise the child for a job well done. Take turns at the turn-taking activity. Continue and do rows two, three and four in the same way.

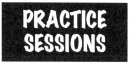

Practice Session 1

Practice the simple sentences using the worksheet, just as you did for the lesson. The child may want to say the sentences on his own, without repeating them after you. Excellent. Actually, you might encourage him to do so. Allow the child to decide whether or not he wishes to select a turn-taking activity or use reinforcers (pennies, poker chips, etc.). Once the child has completed the worksheet, go back and practice any sentences that were difficult for him.

Practice Session 2

Practice sentences using the worksheet. However, this time switch the first two words of the sentences with the other rows. In other words, say each picture in the first row with *I call* instead of *I tell*. In other words, you will say *I call the apple, I call the popsicle, I call the kettle, I call the mule.* Switch *I tell* to another row, such as row two, *I sell* to row three, and *I pull* to row four. You can use any first two words with any row you or the child wishes. Once again, the child can select a turn-taking activity, if he chooses, or do the worksheet alone. Reinforcers (pennies, M & M, etc.) may also be used. Since this is the last time we will be using this worksheet, the child can color in, put a sticker or draw a happy face on each picture for which lllll was correctly said. Do not allow the child to color, put a sticker, or draw a happy face on a picture he said incorrectly. After he completes the sheet go back to the pictures that are not colored or do not have a sticker or happy face. Practice those pictures. Allow the child to color, put a sticker, or draw a happy face on each picture as he succeeds in saying the sentence correctly. Praise him for a job well done.

TROUBLESHOOTING

Some children have difficulty remembering to use lllll or "luh" in sentences. You can help the child get over this difficulty by saying each lllll word of the sentence individually. In other words, you say "I" and the child repeats "I." Next say "call" or "calluh" which the child repeats. Then the child repeats, "the." Last, say the picture name, such as "apple," or "appluh" which the child repeats. Praise the child for a job well done.

Stay on the first picture. This time ask the child to repeat, "I call" or "I calluh." Praise him for a job well done. Now ask him to repeat, "The apple" or " The appluh." Praise him again. Tell the child that this time he will say the whole sentence after you. You slowly say, "I call the apple" or "I calluh the appluh." Ask the child to repeat what you just said. Praise him for a job well done. Complete the first row in this way. Return to Step Two of this lesson once the child repeats each sentence in the first row, in its entirety, using correct lllll in the sentences. Remember to take turns at the turn-taking activity.

If the child has difficulty repeating the entire sentence, stay with "I call," which he repeats, then "the apple," which he repeats. Complete the sheet in this way. Reintroduce the entire sentence, "I call the apple," once you feel the child is ready. The child will be ready to do Step Two of this lesson once he can repeat a simple sentence, in its entirety, for each picture in the first row.

Do not ask or expect the child to use lllll in conversation yet.

LLLLL IN BLENDS

12

GOAL

You will teach the child to use gl, pl, sl, cl, fl, and bl in words.

Note: Not all the blends will be taught in the lesson. Half are taught in the lesson and the other half are taught in Practice Session 1. Or you may want to break this lesson into two therapy sessions. If you do, Practice Session 1 should be treated as another therapy session.

MATERIALS

Worksheets 5 and 6
Turn-taking activity

LESSON TIME

30 minutes

WHAT TO DO

Step One   Review medial words and initial and final simple sentences in Lessons 9, 10, and 11. Praise the child for a job well done. Allow him to take a turn at the activity selected. Move on to Step Two. If the child has difficulty using initial or final lllll in simple sentences or medial words, continue to do those lessons that he is having difficulty with until the child is successful. You may, however, also move on to Step Two, if you feel the child is ready.

⇩   ⇩   ⇩   ⇩   ⇩

Step Two   You will now help the child to use lllll in blends. Look at the first picture on Worksheet 5. As you name this picture you will need to separate the lllll from the rest of the word by a short pause. In other words, instead of saying "clown," say "c," then "lown." Ask the child to say the word with you. Together with the child say "c," and move right into "lown." If this is too difficult for the child, see Troubleshooting.

If the child is successful, move on to the next picture – "clock." Say "c" then "lock." Do the same thing together with the child. For the next word, say the word separating the "c" from the rest of the word with a short pause. Ask the child to repeat what you just said. If he cannot say the word correctly alone, say it together, separating the "c" from the rest of the word. Now ask the child to say the word by himself, just the way you said it together. Follow these steps for the rest of the worksheet:

1. Say the word in a normal fashion. That is, do not separate the first consonant from the rest of the word. Ask the child to name the picture as you did. If he names the picture using a correct lllll, move on to the next picutre and do the same. If he has difficulty producing a clear lllll, move on to #2 below.
2. You say the word separating the first consonant from the rest of the word.
3. The child repeats what you just said, separating the initial consonant from the rest of the word. If he cannot say the word on his own, see #4 below. If he says the word correctly alone, move on to the next picture and repeat #1. You will not need to do #s 4 and 5 below if #1 is easy for the child. Remember to take turns at the trun-taking activity.
4. You and the child say the word together separating the first consonant from the rest of the word.
5. Move on to the next picture and start from #1 again. Remember to take turns at the turn-taking activity.

PRACTICE SESSIONS

Practice lllll in blends using Worksheet 6. Allow the child to decide whether or not he wishes to select a turn-taking activity or use reinforcers (pennies, poker chips, etc.). Before you start, think back to Step Two of this lesson. Was the child able to repeat the lllll in blends? If the answer is yes, the child should be able to repeat these new words without separating the first consonant from the rest of the word. Complete this sheet saying the words as you would do normally.

If necessary, continue to separate the first consonant from the rest of the word when naming these pictures. Try to introduce the unseparated word after three words have been correctly repeated. Ask the child to say the words just the way you say them.

Practice Session 1

Worksheets 5 & 6 will be used for this practice session. Allow the child to decide whether or not he wishes to use a turn-taking activity and/or reinforcers (raisins, poker chips, etc.). Before you start, tell the child that you will be listening for his good lllll. Point to a picture on one of the worksheets. Say the word as you normally would, without separating the first consonant from the rest of the word. Ask the child to say what you just said. Praise the child. He can put a reinforcer on the picture if he said the word correctly. Point to another picture, name it, and ask the child to say what you just said. The child can continue to put reinforcers on the pictures correctly named. A turn at the turn-taking activity can be taken after three or four pictures are named. Remember to praise the child for a job well done.

If the child has difficulty saying a word, you can help him by separating the first consonant from the rest of the word as was done in Step Two.

Practice Session 2

Worksheets 5 & 6 will be used for this session. Allow the child to select a turn-taking activity if he wishes. He may color the pictures, draw a happy face or place a sticker, raisin, penny, etc., on each picture of each worksheet if it was correctly named.

Practice Session 3

Tell the child that today he will point to the pictures. Tell him that you will be listening for his good lllll sound. Ask the child to point to a picture and name it. Praise him for a job well done. If he likes, he may color the picture, or draw a happy face on each picture. Or, if he is using pennies, stickers, etc., allow him to place one on the picture if it was correctly named. Ask the child to point to three more pictures and name each. Praise the child and take turns at the turn-taking activity if one was selected. If the child has difficulty naming the picture, you name it and ask him to say what you said. Do not allow the child to color, draw a happy face, or put a reinforcer on a picture that is difficult for him. Instead, after the child has completed the worksheets, go back to those pictures that are not colored or do not have a sticker, raisin, etc. Ask the child to name those pictures again. He can color, draw a happy face on, or put a reinforcer on each picture named correctly. Remember to praise the child for a job well done.

TROUBLESHOOTING:

Some children have difficulty blending two consonants together. You can help the child by separating the lllll from the rest of the word. Look at the first picture on Worksheet 5. Instead of saying, "clown," you will say "c," which the child repeats, then, "lown," which the child repeats. Praise the child for a job well done. Say each word in the first row in this way – you say the first consonant, the child says the first consonant, you say the rest of the word, the child says the rest of the word. Praise the child for a job well done.

After you and the child have finished the first row, return to Step Two of the lesson. Or, you may choose to do another row, or the entire worksheet, in this way, separating the first consonant from the rest of the word. That is fine. When you feel the child is ready, return to Step Two of the lesson.

Do not ask or expect the child to use lllll in conversation yet.

SENTENCES USING INITIAL, MEDIAL, AND FINAL LLLLL AND LLLLL IN BLENDS

 GOAL

The child will use lllll, in any position, in sentences.

  MATERIALS

Worksheets 7, 8 and 9
Turn-taking activity (optional)

 LESSON TIME

20 minutes

WHAT TO DO

Step One   You and the child should sit next to each other. Look at Worksheet 7. Each picture has writing under it. Tell the child that you will be reading a story together. If he does not yet read, you will read the first sentence under the picture. Read the sentence slowly, with a slight exaggeration of every lllll sound. Ask the child to repeat the sentence you just read. (If the sentence is too long for the child, read part of the sentence. Have the child repeat that portion, then read the next part of the sentence.) If he is a reader, ask him to read the sentence. Remind him to say all his lllll sounds. Listen carefully and make sure each lllll is clearly pronounced. For now, it is better if the child exaggerates the lllll in the sentences. By exaggerating the lllll sounds, the child is able to hear the correct lllll better. The child's ear needs to be trained to recognize it. Up until now the child's ear has accepted the incorrect "w" or "y" sound. Also, the child's tongue must get used to working to produce the new sound. Remember, the tongue was at rest when the child used the "w" or "y".

Listen carefully as the child says the sentences. It is not unusual for children to forget to use the lllll. If the child forgets to use lllll in any word, wait until he has finished the sentence. Tell the child he forgot to use his lllll sound in the word _____. Ask him to repeat the word using his lllll sound. After he has correctly repeat-ed the word, say the same sentence again. Ask the child to repeat what you just said. Every lllll must be clearly pronounced by the child. Praise the child for a job well done. Complete the worksheet with the child, reading no more than one sentence at a time.

⇩   ⇩   ⇩   ⇩   ⇩

Step Two   Look at Worksheet 8 with the child. Do this worksheet just as you did Worksheet 7 in Step One. Remember to frequently praise the child.

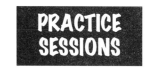

PRACTICE SESSIONS

Sit next to the child. Look at Worksheet 9 with the child. Do this worksheet just as you did Worksheets 7 & 8 of the lesson. Remember to praise the child for a job well done.

Practice Session 1

Sit next to the child. Show the child Worksheets 7, 8 and 9. Ask the child to pick the worksheet he wishes to do first. Do this worksheet just as you did in the lesson. Do the same for the other two worksheets. The child can color in the pictures if he wishes to do so. Remember to praise the child frequently.

Practice Session 2

Sit next to the child. Show the child worksheets 7, 8 and 9. Ask the child questions about the worksheets' stories. Make sure your questions require a sentence answer from the child and not a "yes" or "no" answer. For example, ask questions such as: What happened ...; Why is...; How did ...; etc. You can also elicit speech by saying, "Tell me about...." Watch the child's mouth carefully as he answers. Make sure he uses his correct lllll. If he uses the "w" or "y" sound instead of lllll, tell him on what word he forgot to use his lllll sound. Ask him to say the word again using the lllll sound. Praise him for a job well done. You can begin Lesson 14 after the child completes the worksheets with no lllll errors.

Practice Session 3

Do not ask or expect the child to use lllll in conversation yet.

USING LLLLLL WHILE PLAYING

☆ **GOAL**

The child will use llllll in conversation for a limited period of time in a controlled play environment.

MATERIALS

Cup

Reinforcers:
Small items that can be placed in a cup, such as poker chips, pennies, popcorn, raisins, M&Ms, etc. You will need about 15 of the reinforcers you selected (example: 15 pennies). The child will need to earn a certain number of reinforcers in order to get a reward.

Rewards:
Reward such as a candy bar, ice cream cone, stickers, or any item which will motivate the child. If you use M&Ms, raisins, or other small food as reinforcers, they can be used as the reward. In other words, he gets to eat all the M&Ms he wins. **The reward is given at the end of the lesson**.

Conversational Activities:
You will need an activity that allows you and the child to talk with one another. When playing with the child he should, ideally, dominate the conversation. Avoid doing activities during which you know the child rarely talks. If the child does not talk much while playing, you should try to engage him in conversation about what is happening as you play. Below are examples of activities that are appropriate for this lesson.

- Barbie dolls
- Race cars with gas station or other props you can use to encourage the child to talk while playing.
- Playing school, house, supermarket, astronaut, cowboys, etc. The child may choose to play with or without dolls or action figures.
- Telling a story by looking at pictures in a book is an excellent activity for nonreaders. **If the child is a reader, do not have him read to you.** A reader will see the letter "l" and it will become a clue for him to say his sound correctly. Reading makes this an easier task, similar to what he did in Lesson 13, rather than a conversational task. It is more difficult to remember to use lllll when there are no visual cues.

🕐 **LESSON TIME**

30 minutes

WHAT TO DO

Step One   Allow the child to select an activity along the lines of the examples given under Materials. Tell the child that you will be listening for his good lllll sound as you play together. Tell him that he will earn a chip (or penny or M & M depending on what you have selected) each time he says his good lllll when talking. If he wins three chips, he gets the _____ (name the reward) after the session is over. In other words, the child needs to say lllll correctly a minimum of three times during this entire lesson.

⇩   ⇩   ⇩   ⇩   ⇩

Step Two   The lllll is common enough to appear in *every* sentence one or more times. Listen carefully to the child as he talks. Each time he uses lllll correctly praise him, tell him he gets a chip for using his lllll, and allow him to place one chip in his cup. As you play, give him frequent reminders that you are listening for his good lllll sound when he talks. If the child says an lllll word but forgets to use lllll and uses "w" or "y" instead, do the following:

1. Ask the child to stop playing.
2. Ask the child to look at you.
3. Tell the child that he forgot to use his lllll in the word

_____.
4. Ask the child to say _____ with a good lllll. Praise him after he says the word correctly but do not give him a chip.
5. Remind the child to use his lllll when he talks so that he can get a chip.

If the child uses lllll for words that do not have an lllll sound *see* Troubleshooting
.

It is important to understand that using a new sound in conversation can be a difficult and slow process. This is normal and okay. Your job will be to help the child along so that he gradually uses lllll more frequently. It is of utmost importance to be patient and have realistic expectations. Your goal will be to challenge him without frustrating him or yourself.

PRACTICE SESSIONS

There will be five practice sessions for Lesson Fourteen. It is recommended that the child complete one practice session everyday. Doing a practice session everyday will help the child get used to using lllll in conversation, which will be the goal of the last session, Lesson Fifteen. As you do the practice sessions you will gradually be requiring the child to remember to use lllll more often. You will do this by slowly increasing the number of reinforcers (pennies, chips, etc.) he will need to earn a reward.

You will need reinforcers and a reward. See MATERIALS in the lesson and Appendix B for ideas.

Practice Session 1

Allow the child to select a toy along the lines of that which was selected for the lesson. Tell the child that you will be listening for his good lllll sound while he plays with you. Remind the child that he will win a penny (or whatever reinforcer is selected) each time he says his lllll sound in his words. Tell him that today he will need to win five _____(name the reinforcer) to win a _____(name the reward selected). He gets the reward when the session is over.

Play with the child for about 30 minutes. Follow the instructions under Step Two of the lesson.

You will follow the same instructions for this practice session as you did for Practice Session 1. The child will still need five pennies, or chips, etc., to get a reward.

Practice Session 2

The instructions are the same. However, you will tell the child that this time he will need eight _____(name the reinforcer) in order to get a_____(name the reward) at the end of the session.

Practice Session 3

Practice Session 4

Once again the instructions are the same. Only the number of reinforcers needed for a reward will change. During this session the child will need ten reinforcers in order to win a reward at the end of the session.

Practice Session 5

Same as Practice Session 4.

TROUBLESHOOTING:

Some children overgeneralize using their new sound. In other words, they are not sure which words should have an lllll sound so they use lllll on all words or they randomly use lllll. For example, a child might say, "Lllllbig." You can help the child get over this difficulty by doing the following:

1. Tell the child that not every word has a lllll sound. "Big" does not have a lllll sound. Tell the child we say, "Big."
2. Ask the child to repeat the word correctly: "Big."

Do not ask or expect the child to use lllll in conversation other than during the lesson or practice sessions.

USING LLLLL IN CONVERSATION

 GOAL

The child will learn to use lllll in conversation all the time.

  MATERIALS

- 60 pennies or poker chips of one color
- 10 nickels or poker chips of a different color than was already used
- Two clear cups. One cup should have a picture of a happy face drawn on it.
- Prize that the child will earn. The prize need not be expensive. The child should select the prize. Examples: a special doll or action figure, game, toy, a trip to the movies, clothing, etc. Talk with the parent about the goal of this lesson. The parent should purchase the reward upon completion of the program.

 LESSON TIME

At least one month

WHAT TO DO

Parents using this program should go directly to the Home Program. If you are not the parent, read this entire lesson and familiarize yourself with it. Copy the home program and give it to the parent because he/she will need to complete this lesson at home. Go over the entire lesson with the parent. You will need to see the child once or twice weekly to monitor his progress. During these sessions be prepared to use reinforcers such as chips to reinforce the child's correct production of lllll, as you did in Lesson 14. During each monitoring session, the child will need to earn ten reinforcers to get a reward (sticker, candy, etc) at the end of each session. As the child gets better at using lllll in conversation, you can increase the number of reinforcers needed to earn a treat to a maximum of 15.

There is a certificate at the end of the lesson. Copy, sign, and give the child the certificate after he has successfully completed the home program.

HOME PROGRAM

The home program is the final and most challenging portion of this book. The child will now be expected to use lllll in conversation all the time. This is difficult for a few reasons. First, the child will need to focus on how he talks rather than on what he wants to say. Second, he will need to make a conscious effort to remember to say lllll, learn to catch his errors, and then say the word correctly. Third, he will need to correct his errors when told that he did not say the lllll sound. That means that you will have to interrupt him when he is talking, tell him what word was incorrectly said, and then ask him to say the word correctly.

The home program is challenging for the adult because he/she will need to continually monitor the child, especially the first couple of weeks. Also, you will need to interrupt the child to correct a word and then wait until the child has repeated it correctly.

It is extremely important to be consistent and constant in your monitoring of the child's speech from the outset. It is critical that the momentum of the home program be maintained and that the child remain motivated to correct his speech. If the home program drags on for too long the child will lose his motivation. Once the child ceases to be motivated the home program can extend for months. Focus on the child's conversation and help from you, at the start of the home program, will help the child remember to use the lllll sound more often. As he uses the lllll more, your job will become easier because you will need to correct him less often.

One more important point: always praise the child when he uses lllll without any help from you. Praise lets the child know you are listening, you care, and that he succeeded. Remember that praise is a strong motivator.

Step One

Place the 60 pennies in the clear cup without the happy face. Place the 10 nickels next to the cup.

Show the nickels and the cup with the 60 pennies to the child. Tell the child he is going to try to win all the pennies that are in the cup. Tell him that he will win a penny each time he uses his good lllll when he talks. Each time he wins a penny he will put it into the happy face cup. After he wins all the pennies and nickels he will win a prize of his choice.

Ask the child what prize he would like to win. You might want to take a trip to a store so that he can show you what he wants. The prize should be something the child will be motivated to win. As you do Lesson 15 you will be frequently reminding the child what he is working to win. If the child has a picture of what he wants, you can tape the picture on the second cup instead of drawing a happy face on it.

⇩   ⇩   ⇩   ⇩   ⇩

Step Two   It is very important that you monitor the child whenever he is speaking. The lllll occurs frequently in English. The more often you catch and correct the child's errors the faster he will learn to use lllll in conversation. As you start the penny program, realize that the child will use the "w" or "y" sound more often than he uses lllll. This is normal. He will gradually replace the "w" or "y" with lllll as you correct his errors and reinforce his use of lllll with praise and the earning of pennies. Once the child has earned all his pennies he will be ready for Step Three.

If you find it too difficult to monitor the child throughout the entire day, you can start out by correcting or reinforcing correct use of lllll during specific periods, such as during mealtimes, for the first couple of days. Increase your monitoring from meal-times to an entire half-day, for no more than two more days. Your next increase will be to monitor the child throughout as much of the day as possible.

If the child is in preschool or day care for most of the day, speak to the person caring for the child. Tell this person that the child is learning to use his lllll sound in conversation. Give the caretak-er a small notebook. Ask her to watch the child when he talks. Whenever she hears and sees him using his correct lllll she should praise him and record his using lllll by drawing star in the note-book for each time he used lllll. If the child used lllll five times, then the notebook should have five stars drawn in it. When you pick the child up, ask the caretaker how the child did using lllll during the day. Look at the small notebook, with the child, and together count the number of stars the caretaker made. Praise the child for using lllll. When you get home, place a penny in the cup for each star earned during the day.

WHAT TO DO WHEN THE CHILD CORRECTLY USES LLLLL

As you begin Lesson 15 you will need to give the child a penny each time he correctly uses lllll, on his own, when talking. As he begins to use lllll more often on his own, you will give him pennies less frequently. In other words, as he gets better at using lllll challenge him subtly by giving him a penny after a few words of correct lllll. As time goes on and he uses lllll more often you will give him a penny only after he has spoken over a period of a couple hours without lapsing into the "w" or "y" sound. As you get down to the last ten pennies, you should be giving him a penny for lllll no more than three times a day. How do you know if you are giving too few or too many pennies a day? The following will help you gauge how well you are challenging the child with the penny program:

> Three to four weeks after starting the penny program the child should have earned 30 to 40 pennies and should be using lllll, in conversation, about 50% of the time.
> Four to six weeks after starting the penny program the child should have earned all the pennies and should be using lllll, in conversation, 80% or more of the time.

It is also very important to praise the child. You can praise the child by saying, "Very good! You remembered to say your lllll sound. You said, '_____' (repeat the lllll word your child said correctly)." The child will enjoy placing the penny in the cup by himself. He will also enjoy looking in the cup to see how many pennies he has. Looking in the cup is a good way for the child to see how he is doing. You can also count the pennies with him every now and then. He will be pleased to count how many pennies he has earned.

WHAT TO DO WHEN THE CHILD DOES NOT SAY LLLLL IN CONVERSATION

As you start the penny program expect that the child may use the "w" or "y" sound more often than he will use his correct lllll. When you hear him use the "w" or "y" say, "You forgot to use your lllll. Let's say _____ (name the word that was incorrectly said) using a good lllll sound." Say the word and ask the child to repeat it correctly (do not give him a penny). Praise the child and say "Remember to say your lllll when you talk so you can win pennies. You don't get pennies when you forget to say lllll."

WHAT TO DO IF THE CHILD PURPOSELY SAYS AN LLLLL WORD AND WANTS A PENNY

The child will be eager to earn pennies. As a result he may approach you and say, out of the blue, a word he knows that contains lllll. He may remind you to give him a penny for saying lllll. Praise him for saying a good lllll. You may give him a penny the first couple of times he does this. After the first couple of times, tell him that from now on he gets a penny only when he is talking, and not for thinking of an lllll word to tell you.

WHAT TO DO IF THE CHILD ATTACHES LLLLL TO WORDS THAT DO NOT HAVE AN LLLLL SOUND

Some children overgeneralize when learning to use their lllll sound. In other words, they are not sure which words have an lllll sound so they use lllll on all words or randomly use lllll. For example, a child might say, "Lllllbig." You can help the child get over this difficulty by doing the following:

1. Tell the child there is no lllll in big. Tell the child we say, "Big."
2. Ask the child to repeat the word correctly: "Big."

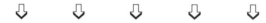

Step Three   This step is designed to help make the child more aware of those times he may still say the "w" or "y" sound for lllll. Once the child has earned all 60 pennies he will be ready to earn nickels. Unlike pennies that could only be won, nickels can be won or lost. In other words, when the child correctly uses lllll for a few hours he earns a nickel and places it in the happy face cup. However, if he says a "w" or "y" sound instead of lllll, he has to take the nickel out of the happy face cup and return it to the original cup.

Congratulate the child for working so hard and winning all his pennies. Tell him that he is almost ready to win his prize. Place ten nickels in the empty penny cup. Remove all the pennies from the happy face cup. Show the nickels to the child and tell him that when all the nickels are in the happy face cup he will get his prize. Tell him he wins a nickel for using his lllll just like when he won pennies. But if he forgets to use his lllll, he has to take a nickel out of the happy face cup and put it back in the other cup. Show him how this works by saying and doing the following:

1. "Let's say you're talking and you use lllll a lot. You win a nickel." (Place a nickel in the happy face cup.)

2. "But let's say you're talking and you forget to use lllll and say 'wion' instead of 'lion.' If you say 'wion,' I have to take one nickel out of the happy face cup and put it back with the other nickels. (Take a nickel out of the happy face cup.) But if you remember to use your lllll again, you can win back the nickel."

3. "Remember to use your lllll so that you don't have to lose any nickels."

4. Write down each lllll word the child incorrectly says. At the end of the day go over the words with the child. Say, "Today you forgot to use your lllll for the words I wrote on this paper. We need to practice these words so that tomorrow you will say them correctly and you will not lose a nickel." Then ask him to say each word correctly five times in a row.

It is normal for the child to lose and earn nickels over the course of a few days. Each time a nickel is lost ask the child to say the word correctly. Remind him to think about using his good lllll so he will not have to lose nickels.

The child should finish the nickels and the lllll program once he uses lllll 100% of the time. Once the child has earned all ten nickels, the person who worked on this program with your child should be told your child is finished. She will give your child a certificate of achievement for completing the program. Once your child receives the certificate, he can have the reward he worked hard to earn.

MAKING SURE THE CHILD CONTINUES TO USE THE LLLLL SOUND

Congratulations to you for having taught the child how to say lllll and the child for having successfully learned to say the lllll sound! Before you put this manual away, however, I would like to leave you with a few suggestions and words of advice regarding the child's newly learned sound.

- First, over the next few days give the child frequent praise for using his good lllll sound. Be generous with praise.
- Second, be on guard for an occasional lapse back to the "w" or "y" sound. If the child slips, bring the error to his attention. Tell him that he forgot to use his lllll when he said _____. Ask him to repeat the word with his" lllll" sound.

If you notice a gradual increase in the use of "w" or "y" for lllll, I suggest that you begin a motivational program to get the child back on track. For instance, tell him that each morning he will get five nickels in his happy face cup. Tell him he will lose a nickel each time he forgets to use his lllll sound. He must have at least one nickel left in his cup at the end of the day to get a reward (such as ice cream, candy, watch a favorite TV program, etc.). After a day or two of getting rewards, reduce the nickels in his happy face cup to three. By reducing the number of nickels, you are requiring him to make fewer errors in order to win a reward at the end of the day. Within a few days the child should be back on track.

Certificate of Achievement

This certifies that

_____

has successfully completed

the "I" Program

on this _____ day of _____

_____

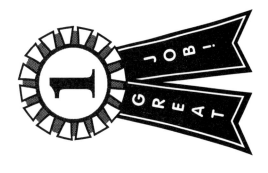

WORKSHEETS

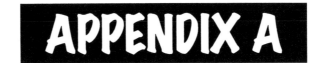

Copy each worksheet as indicated in the appropriate lesson. Since the worksheets will be reused in other lessons, do not discard worksheets until indicated in the lesson.

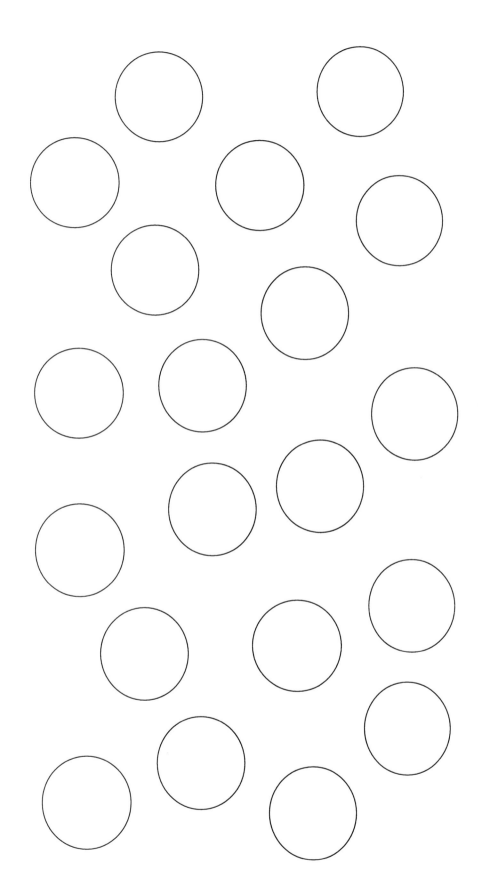

WORKSHEET 2

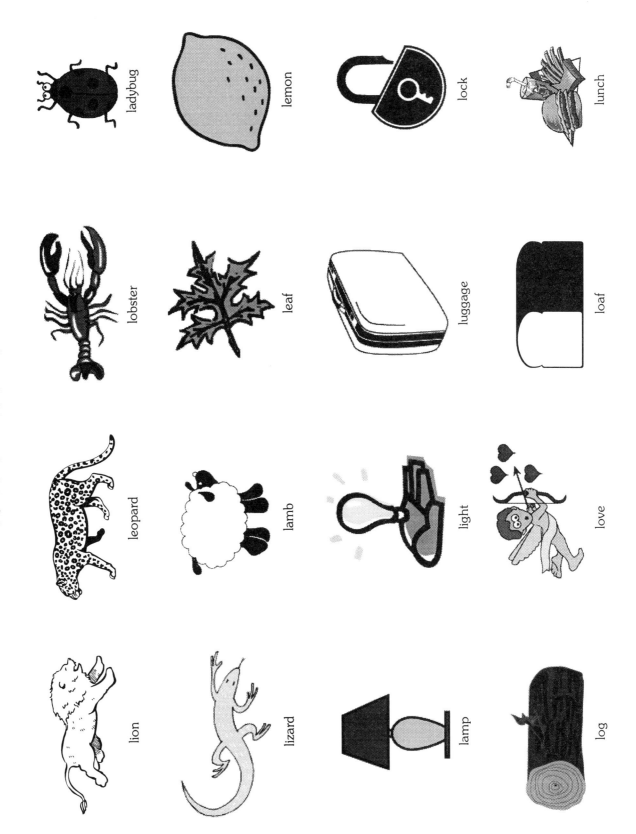

ladybug

lemon

lock

lunch

lobster

leaf

luggage

loaf

leopard

lamb

light

love

lion

lizard

lamp

log

WORKSHEET 3

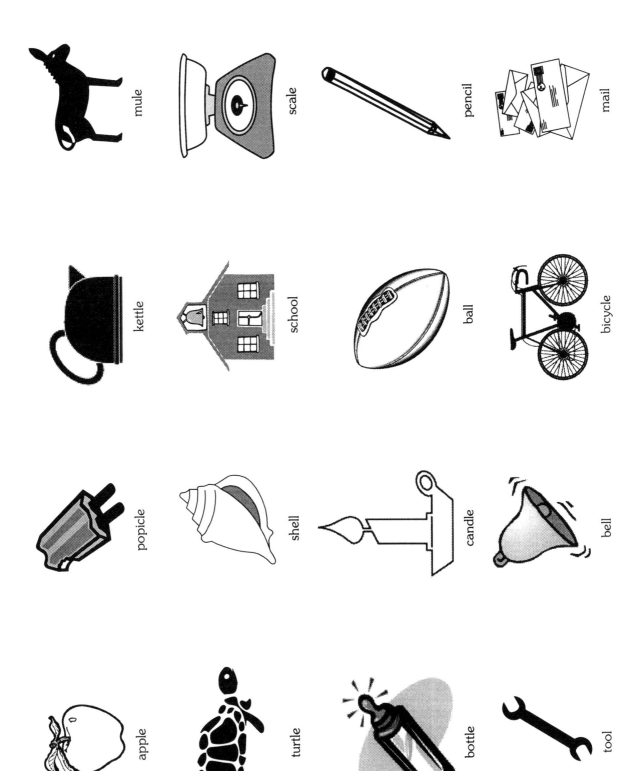

mule

scale

pencil

mail

kettle

school

ball

bicycle

popicle

shell

candle

bell

apple

turtle

bottle

tool

WORKSHEET 4

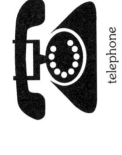 umbrella

 envelope

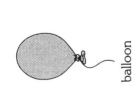 telephone

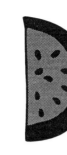 elephant

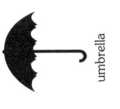 alligator

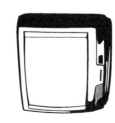 watermelon

 dollar

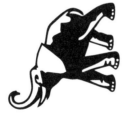 violin

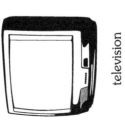 broccoli

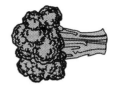 helicopter

 stapler

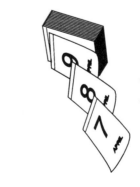 ballet

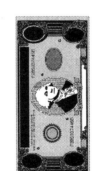 balloon

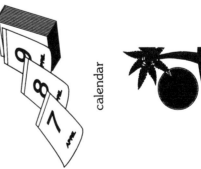 television

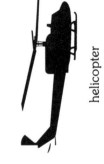 calendar

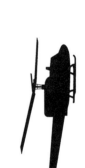 island

75

WORKSHEET 5

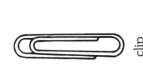

clip

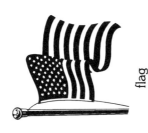

flag

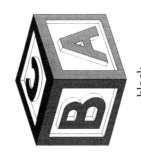

block

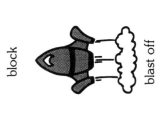

blast off

clover

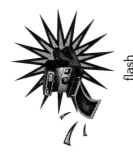

flash

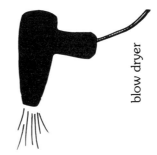

blow dryer

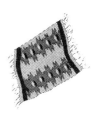

blanket

clock

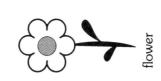

flower

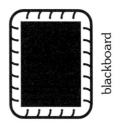

blackboard

blender

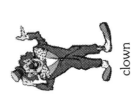

clown

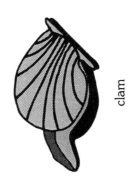

clam

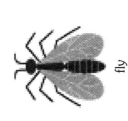

fly

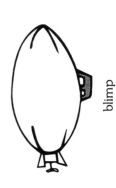

blimp

77

WORKSHEET 6

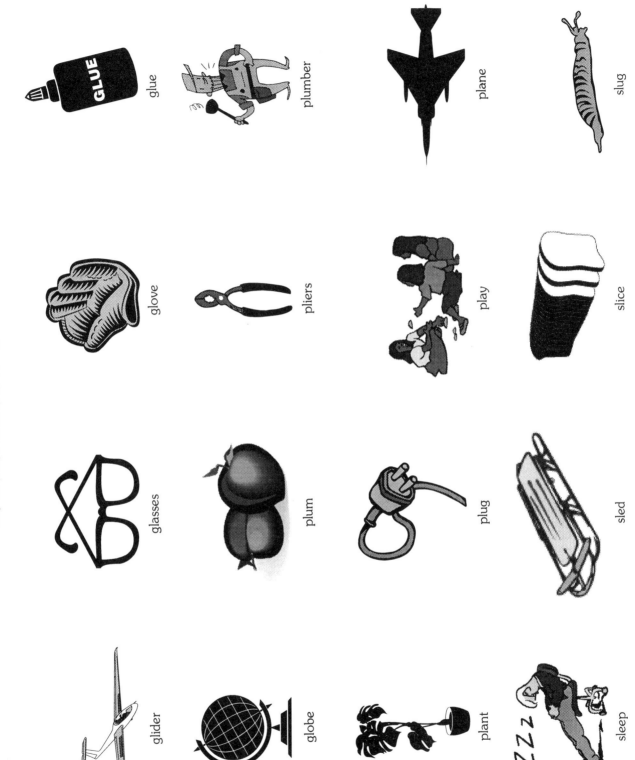

glue

plumber

plane

slug

glove

pliers

play

slice

glasses

plum

plug

sled

glider

globe

plant

sleep

WORKSHEET 7

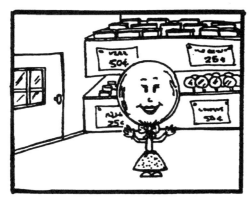

Lena is a lollipop.
She is not too little or too large.

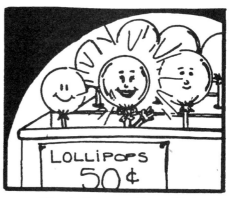

She is the most beautiful
lollipop on the shelf.

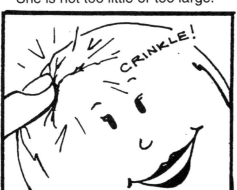

Her yellow wrapper crinkles
when you touch it.

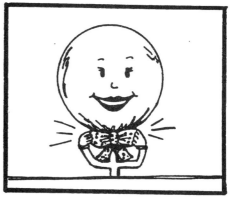

Lena loves her light blue bow.
She wears it around her neck.

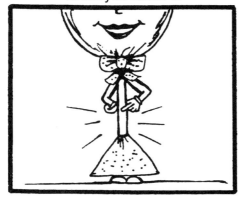

Her stick is a
violet color.

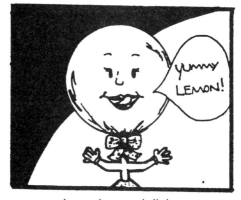

Lena has a delicious
lemon taste.

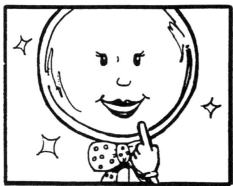

Lena always wears a
big smile.

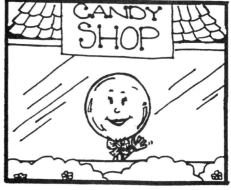

Look for Lena at the candy shop.
She will be looking for you

81

WORKSHEET 8

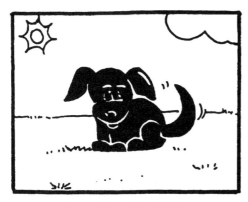

Lucy is a black lab.

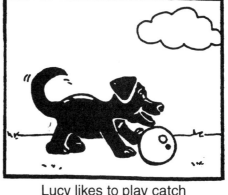

Lucy likes to play catch
with her blue ball.

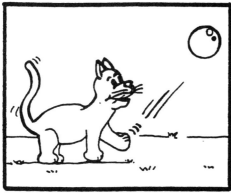

Lola is her pal.
Lola lobs the ball up high.

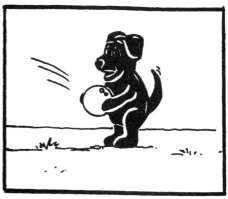

Lucy looks.
She jumps and catches the ball.

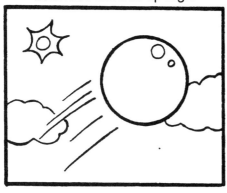

One day, Lola lobbed
the ball very high.

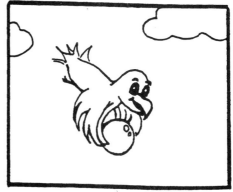

Dolly, the eagle,
caught the ball.

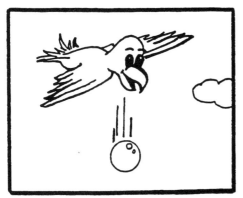

Dolly flew.
Dolly let the ball go.

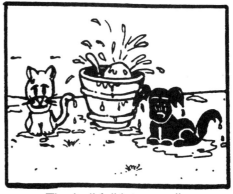

The ball fell into a pail.
Now look at Lucy and Lola.

83

WORKSHEET 9

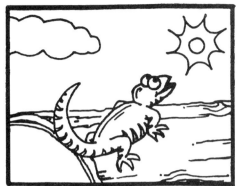

Jello is a lime-green lizard.
His home is an old log.

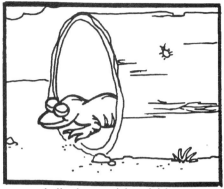

Jello loves his old log.
It is cozy and safe.

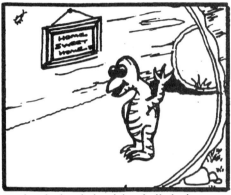

Let's look inside Jello's log.
He has a moss carpet. It is green.

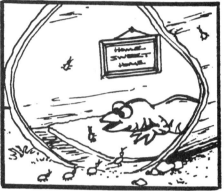

Bugs like his log. Bugs don't like
Jello. He eats them for lunch.

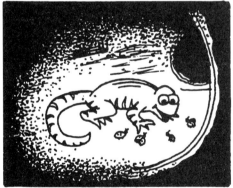

The fireflies light up
Jello's log at night.

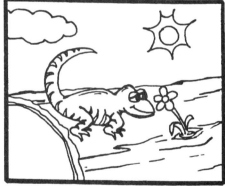

A yellow flower grows on the log.
Jello planted it there last week.

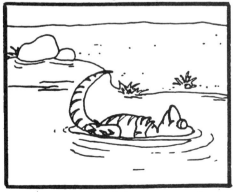

There is a puddle next to the
log. It is Jello's pool.

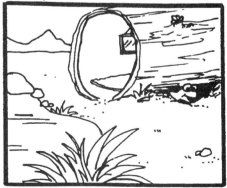

Now Jello is hiding.
Do you know where to look?

85

ACTIVITIES & MATERIALS

GAME TURN-TAKING ACTIVITIES

Games are fun because they allow you and the child to play together by taking turns. Remember that taking a turn is used as a reward for success. For example, the child said lllll in isolation five times, as you asked him to do. He can take a turn. Then you take a turn. Taking a turn should also be a reward for effort even if the goal has not been met. Try to finish the lesson and the turn-taking activity at the same time. As you do the lessons there will be reminders to take turns at the turn-taking activity.

You can also make up your own board games. You will need a large piece of cardboard or poster board and markers or crayons. You draw a scene with a starting point and ending point. Draw a path divided into segments between the start and finish. Game pieces can be buttons, stones, or other small items. You can use dice or make a spinner. Homemade creative games are inexpensive and as much fun as purchased games.

The games listed below are appropriate for children ages four and older and can be found in most toy stores.

Boggle Junior
Bed Bugs
Ants in the Pants
Checkers
Crocodile Dentist
101 Dalmatians
Don't Wake Daddy
Hungry Hungry Hippos
Poppin' Magic
Squiggly Worms
Hi Ho! Cherry-O
Sound Safari
Oops & Downs
Goldilocks and the Three Bears Game
Don't Break the Ice
Animal Crackers Game
Snoopy's Doghouse Game
The Snoopy Game
How Does Your Garden Grow?
Pickup sticks
Marbles

NONGAME TURN-TAKING ACTIVITIES

Nongame activities are completed by the child in segments. In other words, the child does a portion of the activity as a reward for success. For example, if the child has selected Colorforms, he can place three or four colorform pieces on the background as a reward for saying lllll in isolation five times.

Colorforms
Magna Doodle
Etch A Sketch
Perler Beads
Luma Sketch
Tinkertoy
Lincoln Logs
Mr. Mighty Mind
Magna Shapes
Marble Works

CONVERSATIONAL MATERIALS AND ACTIVITIES

Conversational materials and activities are used to stimulate the child to talk. Engage the child in conversation as you play. Allow the child to take on whichever role he chooses (example: mechanic, doctor, dentist, etc.). The child should become involved in playing his part and conversing with you as you play your part. You can find many of the items for the activities around the house. Many can be found as children's play sets at toy stores.

Play beauty partor/barber shop
Play fix-it person
Play farm
Play garage mechanic
Play with Barbie, Ninja Turtles, Batman, etc.
Play restaurant
Play supermarket
Make-believe cooking or baking
Have a tea party
Play birthday party
Play doctor or dentist office
Play secretary
Play police station
Play fire station
Play hospital
Play with the Playmobile figures and sets

NOTES

NOTES

NOTES

NOTES

NOTES